JOINT MOTION
Method of Measuring and Recording

AMERICAN ACADEMY OF ORTHOPAEDIC SURGEONS

Approved by appointed committees of the following:

1 — American Orthopaedic Association
2 — Australian Orthopaedic Association
3 — British Orthopaedic Association
4 — Canadian Orthopaedic Association
5 — New Zealand Orthopaedic Association
6 — South African Orthopaedic Association

Churchill Livingstone

EDINBURGH LONDON MELBOURNE AND NEW YORK 1988

CHURCHHILL LIVINGSTONE
Medical Division of Longman Group UK Limited

Distributed in the United States of America by Churchill
Livingstone Inc., 1560 Broadway, New York, N.Y. 10036,
and by associated companies, branches and representatives
throughout the world.

Originally published by American Academy of Orthopaedic
Surgeons in 1965 and reprinted with their kind permission
by the British Orthopaedic Association 1966

First reprint	1966	Ninth reprint	1978
Second reprint	1966	Tenth reprint	1980
Third reprint	1968	Eleventh reprint	1983
Fourth reprint	1969	Twelfth reprint	1986
Fifth reprint	1971	Thirteenth reprint	1988
Sixth reprint	1972	Fourteenth reprint	1991
Seventh reprint	1974		
Eighth reprint	1976		

ISBN 0-443-00270-3

Produced by Longman Singapore Publishers (Pte) Ltd
Printed in Singapore

CONTENTS

JOINT MOTION
Method of Measuring
and Recording

INTRODUCTION

The Executive Committee of the American Academy of Orthopaedic Surgeons appointed this committee in 1959 to study Joint Motion. This appointment was prompted by increasing requests from members of the Academy for a single, standard, "agreed-upon" method of measuring and recording joint motion.

In 1961, the method as proposed by our Committee was accepted in principle by the Executive Committee of the Academy. It was their recommendation that this method be sent to all members of the American Academy of Orthopaedic Surgeons and the American Orthopaedic Association as a trial pamphlet, for their comments, criticisms and suggestions. Pamphlets were also sent to the Orthopaedic Associations of New Zealand, Australia, South Africa, Canada and Britain. In 1962, the pamphlet was revised in light of the response of the Academy members, and approved for final publication by the Executive Committee. Subsequently, a joint meeting of representatives of these organizations was held in Vancouver, B.C., in 1964 at which time the principle of the method was unanimously accepted. All corrections, additions and deletions agreed upon at this meeting, have been incorporated in this revision.

The section on the Hand has been produced in co-operation and consultation with the American Society for Surgery of the Hand.

Our Committee wishes to thank the members of the Academy who responded by letter and personal communication to the trial booklet. With their help we have been able to make this a more representative method. It also expresses appreciation to orthopaedic associations of the English speaking countries for their interest and help in standardizing the method of describing joint motion. The Committee wishes to thank, also, Mrs. Edith Tagrin, medical artist of the Massachusetts General Hospital, who illustrated this pamphlet, for her cooperation and imagination in this work. We are indebted to the various Executive Committees of the Academy with whom we have worked, from the inception of the idea to standardize joint motion, to this final edition.

Prepared and submitted by

MEMBERS OF THE COMMITTEE FOR THE STUDY OF JOINT MOTION

Charles V. Heck, M.D., Chicago, Illinois

Irvin E. Hendryson, M.D., Denver, Colorado

Carter R. Rowe, M.D., Boston, Massachusetts, CHAIRMAN

THE PRINCIPLES

1. The method of measuring and recording joint motion, as used in this booklet, is based on the principles of the Neutral Zero Method as described by Cave and Roberts in 1936 (2).

2. In this method, all motions of a joint are measured from defined Zero Starting Positions. Thus, the degrees of motion of a joint are added in the direction the joint moves from the Zero Starting Position.

3. The extended "anatomical position" of an extremity is, therefore, accepted as zero degrees, rather than 180 degrees.

4. This method will eliminate the confusion that has existed in the past of measuring joint motions from various starting positions.

5. The motion of the extremity being examined should be compared to that of the opposite extremity. The difference may be expressed in degrees of motion as compared to the opposite extremity, or, in percentages of loss of motion in comparison with the opposite extremity.

6. If the opposite extremity is not present, the motion should be compared to the average motion of an individual of similar age and physical build. Likewise, motions of the spine may be compared to individuals of similar age and physique.

7. Motions are described as active or passive.

8. A distinction is made between the terms "extension" and "hyperextension". Extension is used when the motion opposite to flexion, at the Zero Starting Position, is a

natural motion. This is present in the wrists and shoulder joints. If, however, the motion opposite to flexion at the Zero Starting Position is an unnatural one, such as that of the elbow or knees, it is referred to as hyperextension.

9. Limitation of joint motion is simply described. (Pg. 10).

10. The motion of a joint may be painful. Every effort should be made by the examiner to be gentle. A more accurate estimate of motion may be obtained if the extremity is examined in the position of greatest comfort to the patient.

11. Ankylosis is accepted as the complete loss of motion of a joint.

12. The use of a goniometer is optional, and should be used according to the surgeon's discretion. (Pg. 8).

13. The recording of joint motion should be accurately and clearly tabulated by the examiner. (Pg. 81).

14. A table of average, or normal, ranges of motion is given. These figures must be considered as general estimates, rather than specific standards. (Pg. 82).

TYPES OF JOINT MOTION

Joint motion may be divided
into three general types:

(1) The "one plane (or degree) freedom" of motion, or the true hinge joint, has natural motion in one direction only from the Zero Starting Position. Flexion is motion away from the Zero position and extension is the return motion to the Zero Starting Position. The elbow and knee are examples of hinge joints. As the motion opposite to flexion at the Zero Starting Position is an unnatural one, it is referred to as HYPEREXTENSION.

(2) The "two plane (or degree) freedom" of motion are joints with natural motion in two planes originating from the Zero Starting Position, such as flexion, extension, abduction and adduction (or radial and ulnar and deviation). The wrist is an example of this type of motion.

(3) The "ball and socket" joint consists of three dimensional, compound, or rotatory motion. The hip and shoulder are typical of this type of motion. Three dimensional motion is very complex, and can be analyzed geometrically in "envelopes of compound motion". (10)

USE OF THE GONIOMETER

(1) The goniometer may prove useful in measuring joint motion.

(2) Today many standard goniometers are made which measure a straight line (or the position of the extended extremity) both as zero degrees, and as 180 degrees. This is accomplished by means of double lines of figures, or two indicators on the arm. Examples of these are shown on the opposite page.

(3) When the landmarks of an extremity are definite, the use of the goniometer may be accurate. However, when the bony landmarks are not definite due to excess soft tissue coverage, or other causes, the goniometer may give inaccurate information. In these instances, an experienced surgeon may estimate the angle of motion more accurately without the use of a goniometer.

(4) Therefore, the use of the goniometer should be elective, and used according to the surgeon's discretion.

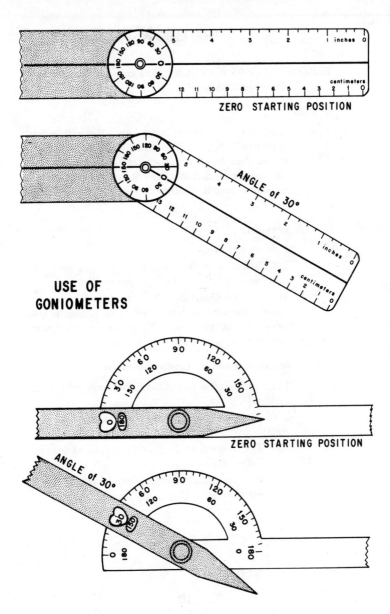

ZERO STARTING POSITION

ANGLE of 30°

USE OF
GONIOMETERS

ZERO STARTING POSITION

ANGLE of 30°

THE ELBOW

ZERO STARTING POSITION: The extended straight arm (zero degrees).

Motions:

The elbow is a typical hinge joint. Natural motion is present in flexion. The opposite motion to flexion, to the Zero Starting Position, is EXTENSION. As the motion beyond the Zero Starting Position is an unnatural one, it is referred to as HYPEREXTENSION.

Fig. A Flexion:

Zero to 150 degrees.

EXTENSION: 150 degrees to Zero (from the angle of greatest flexion to the Zero position).

HYPEREXTENSION: This is measured in degrees beyond the zero starting point. This motion is not present in all individuals. When it is present, it may vary from 5 to 15 degrees.

Fig. B Measurement of Limited Motion:

(The unshaded area indicates the range of limited motion.)

Limited motion may be expressed in the following ways:

(1) The elbow flexes from 30 degrees to 90 degrees.
    (30 → 90)

(2) The elbow has a flexion deformity of 30 degrees with further flexion to 90 degrees.

THE ELBOW

Fig. A FLEXION and HYPEREXTENSION

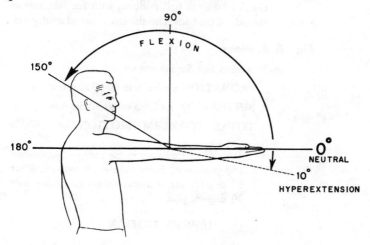

Fig. B MEASUREMENT of LIMITED MOTION

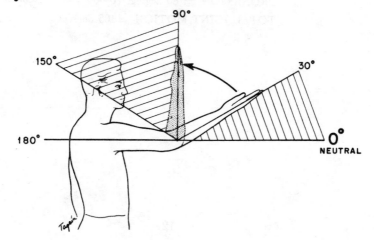

THE FOREARM

ZERO STARTING POSITION: The vertical upright position, or "thumbs up" position, with the forearms at the side of the body, and the elbow flexed 90 degrees.

Fig. A Motions:

Pronation and Supination =

PRONATION = Zero to 80-90 degrees

SUPINATION = Zero to 80-90 degrees

TOTAL FOREARM MOTION = 160-180 degrees

Individuals may vary in the range of supination and pronation. Some individuals may reach the 90 degrees arc, whereas others may have only 70 degrees plus.

LIMITED MOTION

Fig. B Limited motion is simply expressed:

SUPINATION = 45 degrees (0→45°)

PRONATION = 60 degrees (0→60°)

TOTAL JOINT MOTION = 105 degrees

THE FOREARM (Elbow and Wrist)

Fig. A PRONATION and SUPINATION

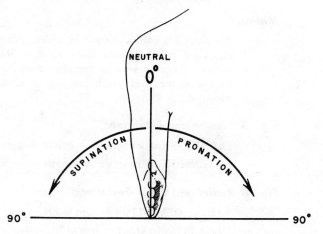

Fig. B MEASUREMENT of LIMITED MOTION

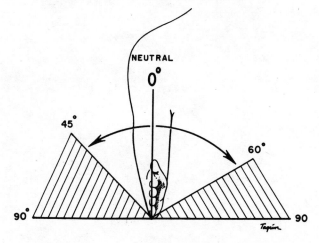

C

THE WRIST

ZERO STARTING POSITION: The extended wrist in line
with the forearm.

Motions:

The wrist has natural motion in flexion, extension,
ulnar and radial deviation from the Zero Starting
position. There is some degree of rotatory circumduction at the wrist which can not be accurately
measured.

Fig. A Flexion and Extension:

FLEXION: (palmar flexion) = zero to 80 degrees ±

EXTENSION (dorsiflexion = zero to 70 degrees ±

Fig. B Radial and Ulnar Deviation:

RADIAL DEVIATION = zero to 20 degrees

ULNAR DEVIATION = zero to 30 degrees

Ulnar deviation is usually measured with the
wrist in pronation. When measured in supination, there is some increase in ulnar deviation.

THE WRIST

Fig. A FLEXION and EXTENSION

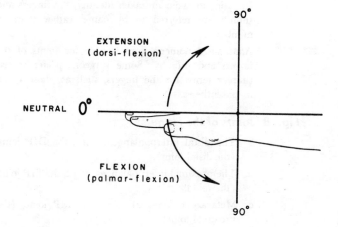

EXTENSION
(dorsi-flexion)

NEUTRAL 0°

FLEXION
(palmar-flexion)

90°

90°

Fig. B RADIAL and ULNAR DEVIATION

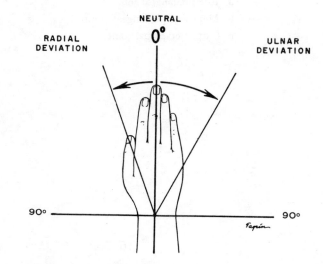

NEUTRAL
0°

RADIAL
DEVIATION

ULNAR
DEVIATION

90°

90°

THE HAND

Fig. A Nomenclature:

In order to avoid mistaken identity, the fingers and thumb are referred to by name, rather than by number.

Anatomical nomenclature is used for joints of the fingers and thumbs. Some surgeons prefer to use simpler terms for the fingers, such as, those noted in parentheses.

Fig. B Joints of the Fingers:

a. The distal interphalangeal joint, the DIP joint, (the distal joint).

b. The proximal interphalangeal joint, the PIP joint, (the middle joint).

c. Metacarpophalangeal joint, the MP joint, (the proximal joint).

Fig. C Joints of the Thumb:

a. Interphalangeal joint

b. Metacarpophalangeal joint

c. Carpometacarpal joint

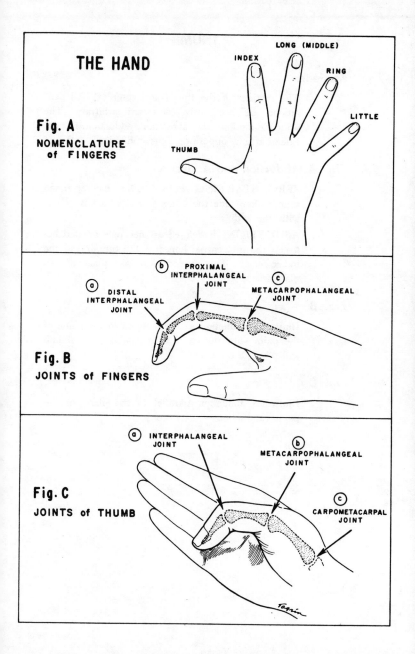

THE HAND

Fig. A
NOMENCLATURE
of FINGERS

INDEX
LONG (MIDDLE)
RING
LITTLE
THUMB

Fig. B
JOINTS of FINGERS

ⓐ DISTAL INTERPHALANGEAL JOINT
ⓑ PROXIMAL INTERPHALANGEAL JOINT
ⓒ METACARPOPHALANGEAL JOINT

Fig. C
JOINTS of THUMB

ⓐ INTERPHALANGEAL JOINT
ⓑ METACARPOPHALANGEAL JOINT
ⓒ CARPOMETACARPAL JOINT

THUMB

Motions:

The motions of the thumb are complex. All definitions are necessarily somewhat arbitrary. The principle motions are: abduction, adduction, flexion, extension and opposition (circumduction).

Fig. A Abduction and Adduction:

ZERO STARTING POSITION: the extended thumb along side the index finger, which is in line with the radius.

ABDUCTION: is defined as the angle created between the metacarpal bones of the thumb and the index finger. This motion may take place in two planes.

Fig. B

Illustrates abduction at right angles to the plane of the palm with the hand in supination, the thumb will point to the ceiling.

Fig. C

Illustrates abduction parallel to the plane of the palm (abduction — extension).

THE THUMB (CIRCUMDUCTION AND ABDUCTION)

Fig. A ZERO STARTING POSITION

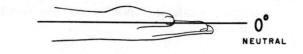

0°
NEUTRAL

Fig. B CIRCUMDUCTION at right angle to the plane of the palm.

90°

0°
NEUTRAL

Fig. C EXTENSION parallel to the plane of the palm.

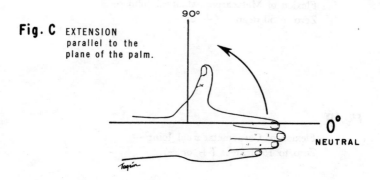

90°

0°
NEUTRAL

THUMB

FLEXION

Fig. A

ZERO STARTING POSITION: The extended thumb.

Fig. B

Flexion of the Interphalangeal Joint —
Zero to 80 degrees (+ or —).

Fig. C

Flexion of Metacarpophalangeal Joint —
Zero to 50 degrees (+ or —).

Fig. D

Flexion of Carpometacarpal Joint —
Zero to 15 degrees (+ or —).

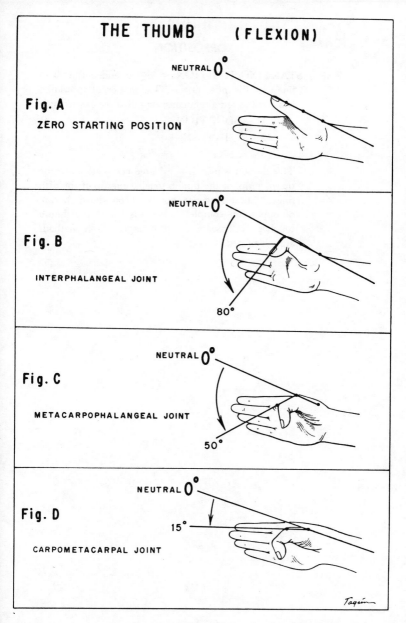

THE THUMB (FLEXION)

Fig. A
ZERO STARTING POSITION

NEUTRAL 0°

Fig. B
INTERPHALANGEAL JOINT

NEUTRAL 0°

80°

Fig. C
METACARPOPHALANGEAL JOINT

NEUTRAL 0°

50°

Fig. D
CARPOMETACARPAL JOINT

NEUTRAL 0°

15°

D

THUMB

OPPOSITION

ZERO STARTING POSITION = the extended thumb in line with the index fingers. The motion of opposition is a composite motion consisting of three elements:

  (1) ABDUCTION
  (2) ROTATION
  (3) FLEXION

This motion is usually considered complete when the tip, or pulp, of the thumb touches the tip of the fifth finger. Some surgeons, however, considered the arc of opposition complete when the tip of the thumb touches the base of the fifth finger. Both methods are illustrated.

THE THUMB — OPPOSITION
COMPOSITE of THREE MOTIONS

ZERO STARTING POSITION

① ABDUCTION

② ROTATION

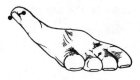

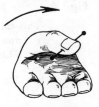

③ and FLEXION

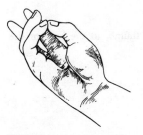

OR

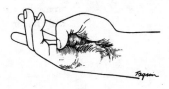

FLEXION TO TIP OF
LITTLE FINGER

FLEXION TO BASE OF
LITTLE FINGER

THUMB
MEASUREMENT OF OPPOSITION

Fig. A

This can be measured in centimeters or inches:
from the tip of the thumb to the top of the
fifth finger, or,

Fig. B

from the tip of the thumb, to the base of the
fifth finger.

THE THUMB
MEASUREMENT of LIMITATION of OPPOSITION

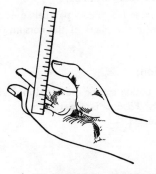

Fig. A   **BY DISTANCE BETWEEN THUMB NAIL AND TOP OF LITTLE FINGER**

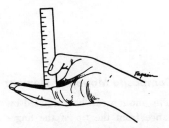

Fig. B   **BY DISTANCE BETWEEN THUMB AND BASE OF LITTLE FINGER**

(ADVICE—"USE 5th FINGER WHEN PRESENT".)

FINGERS

FLEXION

ZERO STARTING POSITION:

> The extended fingers parallel to each other, and in line with the plane of the dorsum of the hand and wrist.

Fig. A Flexion:

> This motion can be estimated in degrees, or in centimeters. Flexion is a natural motion in all joints of the fingers.

Fig. B Composite Motion of Flexion:

> This motion can be estimated by a ruler, as the distance from the tip of the finger (indicate 1. midpoint of pad, 2. nail edge) to the:
> - a. distal palmar crease (this measures flexion of the middle and distal joints)
> - b. proximal palmar crease (this measures the distal, middle and proximal joints of the fingers)

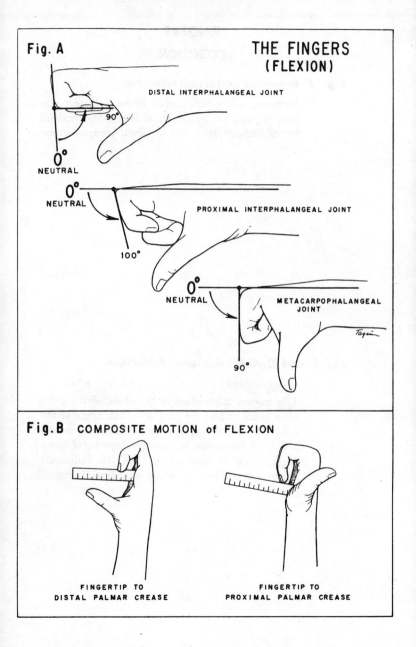

Fig. A
THE FINGERS
(FLEXION)

DISTAL INTERPHALANGEAL JOINT

90°

0°
NEUTRAL

0°
NEUTRAL

PROXIMAL INTERPHALANGEAL JOINT

100°

0°
NEUTRAL

METACARPOPHALANGEAL JOINT

90°

Fig.B COMPOSITE MOTION of FLEXION

FINGERTIP TO
DISTAL PALMAR CREASE

FINGERTIP TO
PROXIMAL PALMAR CREASE

FINGERS

EXTENSION

Fig. A Extension and Hyperextension:

Extension is a natural motion at the metacarpophalangeal joint, but an unnatural one in the proximal interphalangeal joint and the distal interphalangeal joint.

Fig. B and C Abduction and Adduction:

(Finger spread)

This motion takes place in the plane of the palm away from, and to, the long or middle finger of the hand. This can be indicated in centimeters or inches. Spread of fingers can be measured from tip of index finger to tip of little finger. (Fig. C). Individual fingers spread from tip to tip of indicated fingers. (Fig. B).

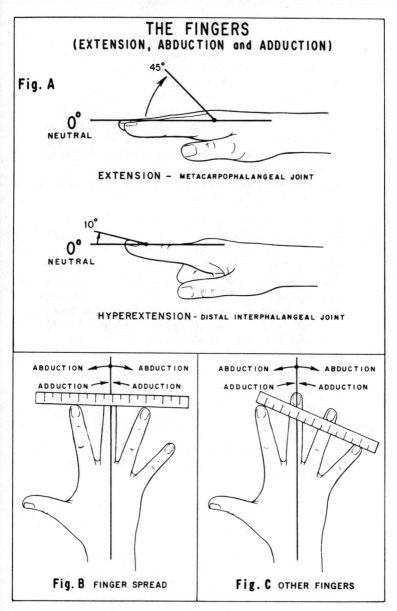

THE FINGERS
(EXTENSION, ABDUCTION and ADDUCTION)

Fig. A

45°

0°
NEUTRAL

EXTENSION – METACARPOPHALANGEAL JOINT

10°

0°
NEUTRAL

HYPEREXTENSION – DISTAL INTERPHALANGEAL JOINT

ABDUCTION ← → ABDUCTION
ADDUCTION → ← ADDUCTION

Fig. B FINGER SPREAD

ABDUCTION ← → ABDUCTION
ADDUCTION → ← ADDUCTION

Fig. C OTHER FINGERS

E

THE SHOULDER

The arm at the shoulder has an almost complete range of global motion. The terms in common usage in the past, such as "abduction", "forward flexion" and "backward extension", have described only the vertical or upward motion of the arm at the shoulder. As pointed out in the initial "trial" pamphlet, there have been no accepted terms to describe horizontal motion of the arm at the shoulder. Unless shoulder motion is described in the horizontal as well as the vertical planes, the position of the arm, in its global range, can not be accurately defined. This has been a source of confusion in shoulder terminology in the past.

The Committee gave much time and thought to this problem, and suggested a solution in the "trial" pamphlet. However, it was not received with sufficient support. Therefore, the Committee has returned to the terminology in common usage, such as "forward flexion", "backward extension" and "abduction" to define vertical motion of the arm. We have, however, proposed the terms "horizontal flexion" and "horizontal extension" to define the horizontal coordinates, and thus make it possible to pin point the position of the arm in all positions.

GLOBAL MOTION of the SHOULDER

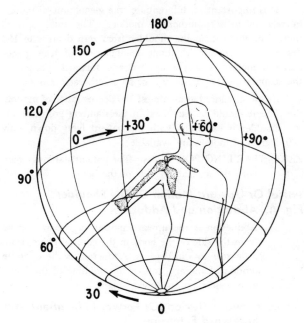

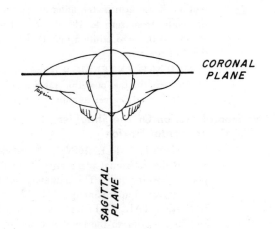

THE SHOULDER

It is important to differentiate true glenohumeral motion in relation to scapulothoracic motion. The total upward motion of the arm at the shoulder from zero degrees to 180 degrees is a smooth rhythmic combination of true glenohumeral motion, plus the upward and forward rotation of the scapula on the chest wall, or scapulothoracic motion.

As the shoulder has an almost 360 degree range of motion, the patient should be examined in the standing position. (If the shoulder is examined with the patient lying down, only 180 degrees of motion are available).

ZERO STARTING POSITION—The patient standing erect, with the arm at the side of the body.

I Vertical Or Upward Motion Of The Shoulder
Fig. A. Abduction and Adduction

Abduction is the upward motion of the arm away from the side of the body in the coronal plane, from 0 degrees to 180 degrees. Adduction is the opposite motion of the arm toward the midline of the body, or beyond it in an upward plane.

Fig. B. Forward Flexion (Or Forward Elevation) And Backward Extension

FORWARD FLEXION is the forward upward motion of the arm in the anterior saggital plane of the body, from zero to 180 degrees. The opposite motion to the zero position may be termed "depression" of the arm.

BACKWARD EXTENSION is the upward motion of the arm in the posterior saggital plane of the body from zero degrees to approximately 60 degrees.

II Horizontal Motion Of The Shoulder
Fig. C. Horizontal Flexion

HORIZONTAL FLEXION is the motion of the arm in the horizontal plane anterior to the coronal plane across the body. This motion is measured from zero degrees to approximately 130°-135°.

HORIZONTAL EXTENSION is the horizontal motion posterior to the coronal plane of the body.

32

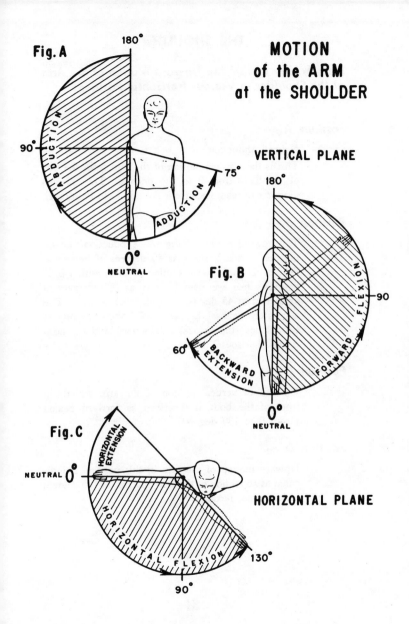

Fig. A

180°

90°

ABDUCTION

75°

ADDUCTION

0°
NEUTRAL

MOTION
of the ARM
at the SHOULDER

VERTICAL PLANE

180°

Fig. B

90

60°

BACKWARD
EXTENSION

FORWARD
FLEXION

0°
NEUTRAL

Fig. C

HORIZONTAL
EXTENSION

NEUTRAL 0°

HORIZONTAL
FLEXION

HORIZONTAL PLANE

130°

90°

THE SHOULDER

Terminology Identifying Upward Motion of the Arm at the Shoulder in Various Horizontal Positions:

Position A —

Neutral Abduction

This is the upward motion of the arm from the side of the body from 0 to 180 degrees. This upward motion can take place from Position G to Position C.

Position B —

The upward motion of the arm (abduction) in this position is taking place at 45 degrees of horizontal flexion. If the upward motion at this position is 90 degrees, then we describe this as "90 degrees of abduction at 45 degrees of horizontal flexion". This accurately defines the position of the extremity in two planes—the vertical (abduction) and the horizontal (horizontal flexion).

Position C —

Upward or vertical motion of the arm directly in front of the body is described as forward flexion (from 0 to 180 degrees).

Position D —

Upward motion of the arm in this position is indicated as adduction of the arm upward, at 135 degrees of horizontal flexion.

THE SHOULDER

TERMINOLOGY IDENTIFYING UPWARD MOTION
OF THE ARM IN VARIOUS HORIZONTAL POSITIONS

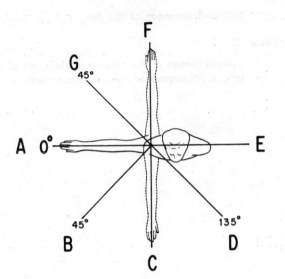

POSITION

A = Neutral abduction

B = Abduction in 45° of horizontal flexion

C = Forward flexion

D = Adduction in 135° of horizontal flexion

E = Neutral adduction

F = Backward extension

G = Abduction in 45° of horizontal extension

F

THE SHOULDER

Position E —

Neutral Adduction of the Arm.

Position F —

Backward Extension of the Arm.

Position G —

Upward motion at this position, is abduction of the arm, at 45 degrees of horizontal extension.

THE SHOULDER

TERMINOLOGY IDENTIFYING UPWARD MOTION OF THE ARM IN VARIOUS HORIZONTAL POSITIONS

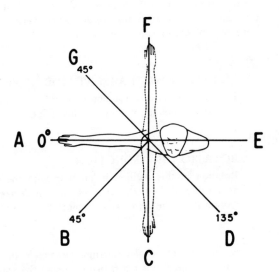

POSITION **A** = Neutral abduction

B = Abduction in 45° of horizontal flexion

C = Forward flexion

D = Adduction in 135° of horizontal flexion

E = Neutral adduction

F = Backward extension

G = Abduction in 45° of horizontal extension

THE SHOULDER

ROTATION

NEUTRAL POSITION:

It is customary to measure rotation of the shoulder in two positions. One with the arm at the side of the body, the second position in 90 degrees of abduction. Rotation can also be measured in any position where vertical and horizontal planes or coordinates cross.

Fig. A

ROTATION WITH ARM AT SIDE OF BODY:
Inward and outward rotation is recorded in degrees of motion from the neutral starting point.

Fig. B

ROTATION IN ABDUCTION:
Rotation in this position is less than with the arm at the side of the body. It is recorded in degrees of motion from the zero starting point.

Fig. C

A clinical method of estimating function is the distance the fingertips reach in relation to the scapula or the base of the neck.

THE SHOULDER (ROTATION)

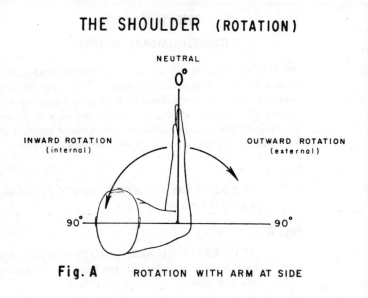

NEUTRAL

0°

INWARD ROTATION
(internal)

OUTWARD ROTATION
(external)

90°   90°

Fig. A   ROTATION WITH ARM AT SIDE

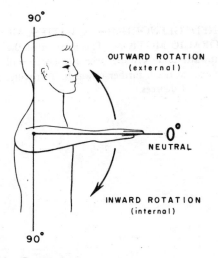

90°

OUTWARD ROTATION
(external)

0°
NEUTRAL

INWARD ROTATION
(internal)

90°

Fig. B ROTATION IN ABDUCTION

Fig. C
INTERNAL ROTATION
POSTERIORLY

THE SHOULDER

GLENOHUMERAL MOTION

It is important to differentiate true glenohumeral motion in relation to scapulothoracic motion. The total upward motion of the arm at the shoulder from zero degrees to 180 degrees is a smooth rhythmic combination of true glenohumeral motion, plus the upward and forward rotation of the scapula on the chest wall, or scapulothoracic motion.

Fig. A

THE NEUTRAL STARTING POSITION with the arm at the side of the body.

Fig. B

TRUE GLENOHUMERAL MOTION is estimated by fixing the scapula with the hand, and elevating the arm passively with the other hand.

Fig. C

"COMBINED" GLENOHUMERAL WITH SCAPULOTHORACIC MOTION. The rotation of the scapula upward and forward over the chest wall allows the arm to reach further upwards. Normally, the range is 180 degrees.

THE SHOULDER (GLENOHUMERAL MOTION)

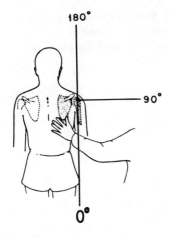

Fig. A NEUTRAL

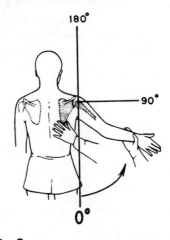

Fig. B RANGE OF TRUE
GLENOHUMERAL MOTION

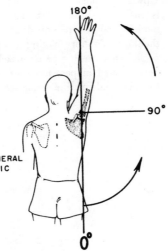

Fig. C

"COMBINED" GLENOHUMERAL
AND SCAPULOTHORACIC
MOTION

MOTIONS OF THE SHOULDER GIRDLE

Fig. A Flexion and Extension

Forward flexion and backward extension of the shoulder girdle are measured in degrees from the neutral starting position. This is primary motion of the scapula and the clavicle.

Fig. B Elevation

Upward motion of the shoulder girdle in elevation is measured in degrees. The opposite downward motion may be described as "depression" of the shoulder. Rotatory motion in the shoulder girdle is possible but can not be accurately measured. It can be estimated in percentage of motion as compared to individuals of similar age and physique.

MOTION of the SHOULDER GIRDLE

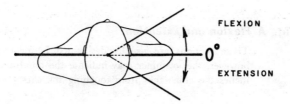

FLEXION

0°

EXTENSION

Fig. A

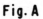

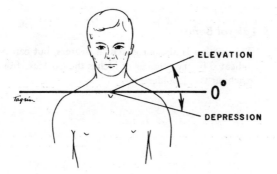

ELEVATION

0°

DEPRESSION

Fig. B

THE CERVICAL SPINE

ZERO STARTING POSITION: The correct standing, or sitting position.

Fig. A Flexion and Extension:

These motions are usually designated by degrees,
however, the examiner may indicate the number of
inches the chin lacks from touching the chest.

Fig. B Lateral Bend:

This motion is also measured in degrees, but can be
indicated by the number of inches the ear lacks from
reaching the shoulder.

Fig. C Rotation:

This is estimated in degrees from the neutral position,
or in percentages of motion, as compared to individuals of similar age and physical build.

THE CERVICAL SPINE

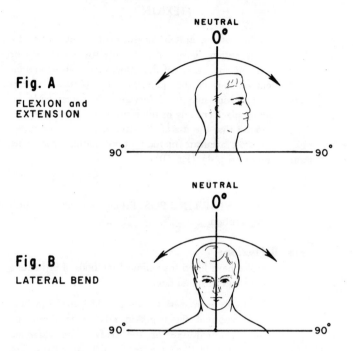

Fig. A

FLEXION and
EXTENSION

NEUTRAL
0°

90°   90°

NEUTRAL
0°

Fig. B

LATERAL BEND

90°   90°

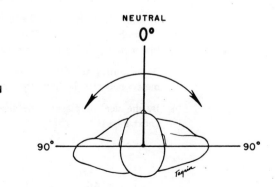

NEUTRAL
0°

Fig. C

ROTATION

90°   90°

THE THORACIC AND LUMBAR SPINE
FLEXION

It is difficult to accurately measure true spine motion by physical examination. This is due to soft tissue coverage of the spine, the normal curves of the spine, variations of motion in different sections of the spine, and the presence of hip motion. In fact, one may bend forward 90 degrees with the motion taking place entirely in the hips, and not in the spine. We have found that the use of the steel or plastic tape measure is the most accurate method of estimating true spine motion in flexion (14) (Pg. 50).

Fig. A
ZERO STARTING POSITION: The correct standing position.

Fig. B Flexion:
We have listed four clinical methods of estimating the range of spinal flexion.

1. By measuring the degrees of forward inclination of the trunk in relation to the longitudinal axis of the body. The examiner should "fix" the pelvis with his hands. The loss (or not) of lordosis should also be noted.

2. By indicating the level the fingertips reach along the patient's leg. For instance, fingertips to the patella; or fingertips to midtibia.

3. By measuring the distance in inches or centimeters between the fingertips and the floor.

4. By the steel or plastic tape measure method (next Page).

THE THORACIC AND LUMBAR SPINE (FLEXION)

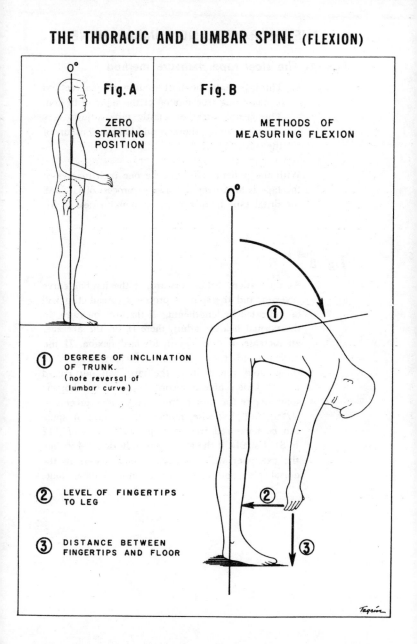

Fig. A

ZERO
STARTING
POSITION

Fig. B

METHODS OF
MEASURING FLEXION

① DEGREES OF INCLINATION
   OF TRUNK.
   (note reversal of
   lumbar curve)

② LEVEL OF FINGERTIPS
   TO LEG

③ DISTANCE BETWEEN
   FINGERTIPS AND FLOOR

THE THORACIC AND LUMBAR SPINE

Fig. A   The steel tape measure method

4. This is perhaps the most accurate clinical method of measuring true motion of the spine in flexion. The flexible steel or plastic tape adjusts very accurately to the thoracic and lumbar contours of the spine. (14).

With the patient standing, the one inch marker of the tape is held over the spinous process of C7, and the distal tape held over the spinous process of S1.

Fig. B

As the patient bends forward, if the lumbar curve reverses, and the spinous processes spread, this will be indicated by lengthening of the tape measure. In the normal healthy adult, there is, on the average, an increase of 4 inches in forward flexion. If the patient bends forward with his back straight (as in rheumatoid spondylitis), the tape will not record motion. One is able to record motion of the thoracic spine per se, by taping from the spinous process of C7 to T12. Likewise, motion of the lumbar spine can be measured from the spinous process of T12 to S1. Usually, if the total spine in flexion is 4 inches the examiner will find that 1 inch occurs in the dorsal spine, and 3 inches occurs in the lumbar spine.

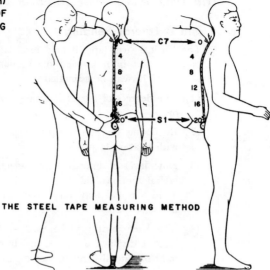

④ THE STEEL TAPE MEASURING METHOD

Fig. A THE PATIENT STANDING ERECT

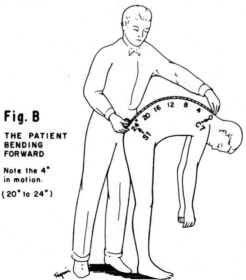

Fig. B

THE PATIENT
BENDING
FORWARD

Note the 4"
in motion.

(20" to 24")

THE THORACIC AND LUMBAR SPINE

Fig. A and B Lateral Bending

The vertical steel tape, if held firmly and straight, may also aid in measuring the motion of lateral bending. This can be estimated in:

(1) The degrees of lateral inclination of the trunk, or,

(2) By noting position of spinous process of C-7 with relation to pelvis.

(3) Note level of lumbar spine reflecting base of lateral motion. This level may be lumbosacral or higher and may vary from right to left in the same patient.

(4) The knee joint may be used as fixed point. Record distance of finger tips from the knee joint on lateral bending (see Figure B).

THE THORACIC AND LUMBAR SPINE
LATERAL BENDING

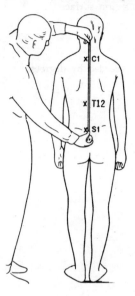

Fig. A

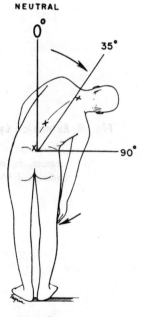

NEUTRAL

0°

35°

90°

Fig. B

THE SPINE

Extension may be recorded with the patient standing, or with the patient lying prone on a firm surface.

Fig. A Extension Standing

The range of extension is recorded by degrees.

Fig. B Extension Lying Prone

The range of motion in this position is measured by degrees, in relation to the position of the spinous process of C-7.

THE THORACIC AND LUMBAR SPINE (EXTENSION)

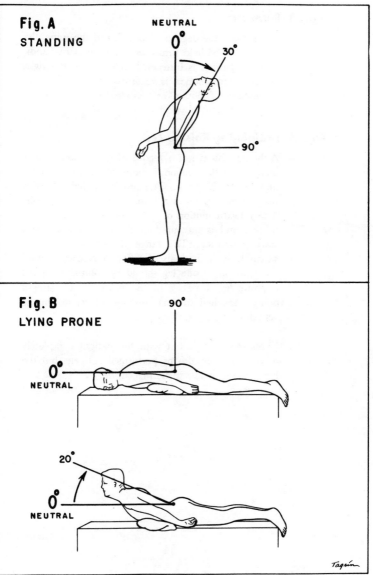

Fig. A
STANDING

NEUTRAL
0°
30°
90°

Fig. B
LYING PRONE

90°
0°
NEUTRAL

20°
0°
NEUTRAL

THE SPINE

Fig. A Rotation

To estimate the degrees of rotation of the spine, the pelvis must be held firmly by the examiner's hands, and the patient is instructed to rotate to the right or left. This motion is recorded in degrees, or in percentages of motion, as compared to individuals of similar age and physical build.

Fig. B Straight Leg Raising Test

Although this is not a record of spine motion, it is included in this section, because of its use in examinations of the back. The test is carried out with the patient supine on a firm, level examining table. The upward motion of the straight leg is a passive motion and is measured in degrees from the zero starting position. This range of motion varies considerably in individuals of different physical builds. The motion of one leg should be compared to the opposite leg. Rotation of the pelvis occurs after a point is reached and may provide an "error" in the actual straight leg raising present.

(This is a passive test with the patient completely relaxed. It may also be performed actively, but the level of rise is apt to be inaccurate.)

Fig. A   THE SPINE — ROTATION

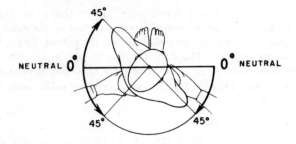

Fig. B   STRAIGHT LEG RAISING TEST (PASSIVE MOTION)

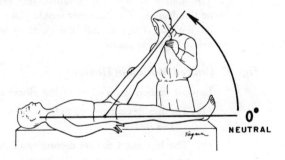

THE HIP

The hip is a "ball and socket" joint. Due to its deeper socket, the range of motion is less than that of the shoulder. Motions of the hip are measured with the patient lying either supine or prone. This simplifies terrminology, as compared to the shoulder, as only one hemisphere of motion is measured at a time. Errors in hip motion occur when pelvis rotation is not noticed.

Fig. A Flexion:

ZERO STARTING POSITION of the right hip: The patient lies supine on a firm, flat surface with the opposite hip held in full flexion. This flattens the lumbar spine and demonstrates a flexion deformity of the hip if it is present.

Fig. B Flexion:

The motion in flexion is recorded from zero to 110 or 120 degrees. The examiner should place one hand on the iliac crest to note the point at which the pelvis begins to rotate.

Fig. C Limited Motion in Flexion:

Limited motion is noted as in the elbow and knee.

(1) The hip flexes from 30 to 90 degrees.
    (30 → 90)

(2) The hip has a flexion deformity of 30 degrees with further flexion to 90 degrees.

THE HIP (FLEXION)

Fig. A ZERO STARTING POSITION

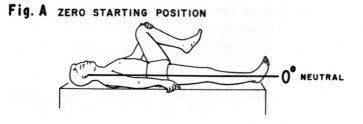

0° NEUTRAL

Fig. B FLEXION

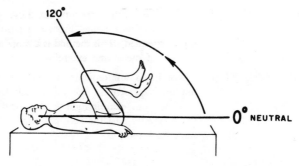

120°

0° NEUTRAL

Fig. C LIMITED MOTION in FLEXION

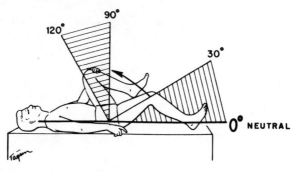

90°

120°

30°

0° NEUTRAL

THE HIP

Fig. A Extension

ZERO STARTING POSITION:

The patient lies prone on a firm, level surface.

Fig. B Extension

The upward motion of the hip is measured in degrees from the Zero Starting Position. Two methods are commonly used:

(a) With the patient face down and a small pillow under the abdomen, the leg is extended with the knee straight or flexed.

(b) With the opposite extremity flexed over the end of the examining table. From this position, the hip is extended. This method is a more accurate method of measuring extension.

(c) There is an anatomical question whether extension is present in the hip at all. Extension as seen from examination is that deviation of the extremity past the zero position and reflects some back motion.

THE HIP (EXTENSION)

Fig. A ZERO STARTING POSITION

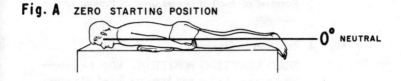

0° NEUTRAL

Fig. B EXTENSION

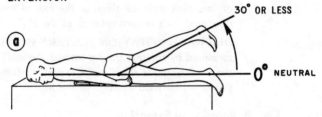

(a)

30° OR LESS

0° NEUTRAL

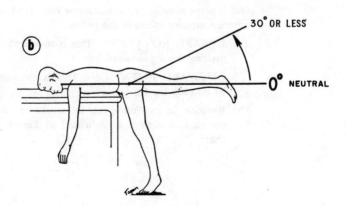

(b)

30° OR LESS

0° NEUTRAL

THE HIP

Rotation:

Rotation of the hip is measured in flexion, and in extension.

Fig. A Rotation in Flexion:

ZERO STARTING POSITION: With the patient lying supine, the hip and knee are flexed 90 degrees each, with the thigh perpendicular to the transverse line across the anterior superior spines of the pelvis.

INWARD ROTATION (INTERNAL): This is measured by rotating the leg away from the midline of the trunk with the thigh as the axis of rotation, thus producing inward rotation of the hip.

OUTWARD ROTATION (EXTERNAL): This is measured by rotating the leg toward the midline of the trunk with the thigh as the axis of rotation, thus producing outward rotation of the hip.

Fig. B Rotation in Extension

ZERO STARTING POSITION: With the patient lying face down, the knee is flexed to 90 degrees and is perpendicular to the transverse line across the anterior superior spines of the pelvis.

(a) INWARD ROTATION: This is measured by rotating the leg outward.

OUTWARD ROTATION: This is measured by rotating the leg inward.

(b) Rotation in extension can be measured with the patient supine, as indicated in Figure B, chart (b).

THE HIP   (ROTATION)

Fig. A ROTATION in FLEXION

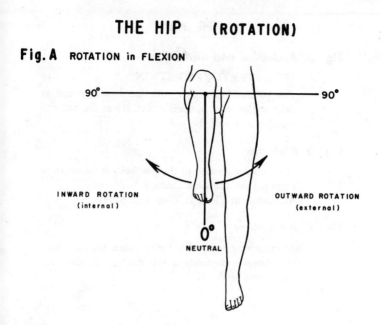

90° — — — 90°

INWARD ROTATION
(internal)

OUTWARD ROTATION
(external)

0°
NEUTRAL

Fig. B ROTATION in EXTENSION

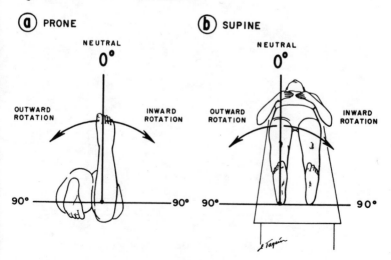

(a) PRONE

NEUTRAL
0°

OUTWARD
ROTATION

INWARD
ROTATION

90° — — — 90°

(b) SUPINE

NEUTRAL
0°

OUTWARD
ROTATION

INWARD
ROTATION

90° — — — 90°

THE HIP

Fig. A *Abduction and Adduction:*

ZERO STARTING POSITION

The patient lies supine with the legs extended at right angles to a transverse line across the anterior superior spines of the pelvis.

Fig. B *Abduction:*

The outward motion of the extremity is measured in degrees from the Zero Starting Position.
Abduction in Flexion: (See next page).

Fig. C *Adduction:*

In measuring adduction, the examiner should elevate the opposite extremity a few degrees, to allow the leg to pass under it.

THE HIP (ABDUCTION and ADDUCTION)

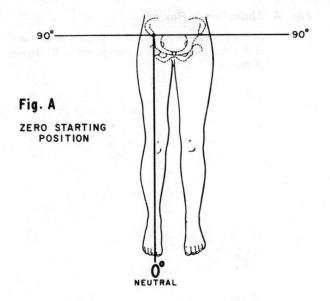

90° ——————————————————— 90°

Fig. A

ZERO STARTING
POSITION

0°
NEUTRAL

Fig. B ABDUCTION

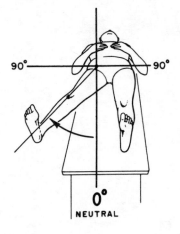

90° 90°

0°
NEUTRAL

Fig. C ADDUCTION

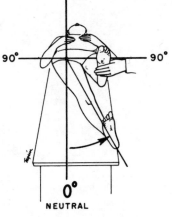

90° 90°

0°
NEUTRAL

Fig. A Abduction in Flexion:

Abduction can be measured in degrees at any level of flexion. Usually, this is carried out in 90 degrees of flexion.

THE HIP

Fig. A   ABDUCTION in FLEXION

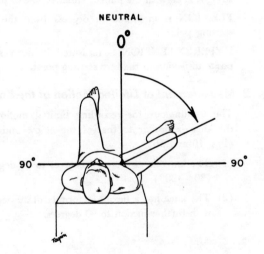

NEUTRAL

0°

90°   90°

KNEE

The knee is considered to be a modified hinge joint, with its primary motion in flexion. The motion opposite to flexion to the zero starting position is extension. As the motion beyond the zero starting position is an unnatural one, it is referred to as hyperextension. There is a small degree of natural rotation of the tibia on the femoral condyle in flexion and extension. This can not be accurately measured. Abnormal lateral motion may be estimated in degrees.

Fig. A Flexion:

ZERO STARTING POSITION: The extended straight knee with the patient either supine or prone.

FLEXION is measured in degrees from the zero starting point.

HYPEREXTENSION is measured in degrees opposite to flexion at the zero starting point.

Fig. B Measurement of Limited Motion of the Knee:

The terminology for recording limited motion of the knee is similar to that of the elbow and hip. (Pgs. 10 and 56).

(1) The knee flexes from 30 degrees to 90 degrees. (30°→90°)

(2) The knee has a flexion deformity of 30 degrees with further flexion to 90 degrees.

THE KNEE

Fig. A FLEXION and HYPEREXTENSION

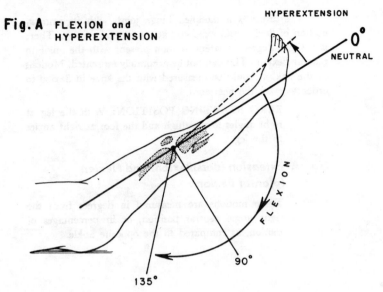

Fig. B MEASUREMENT of LIMITED MOTION

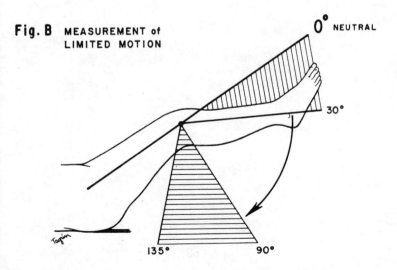

THE ANKLE

The ankle is a modified hinge joint, with its primary motion of flexion and extension at the tibiotalar joint. There is a slight degree of lateral motion present with the ankle in plantar flexion. This can not be accurately estimated. Motions of the ankles should be measured with the knee in flexion in order to relax the heel cord.

> ZERO STARTING POSITION: With the leg at right angles to the thigh and the foot at right angles to the leg.

Fig. A Extension (dorsiflexion) and Flexion (plantar flexion):

> These motions are measured in degrees from the right angle neutral position, or in percentages of motion, as compared to the opposite ankle.

THE ANKLE

Fig. A   FLEXION and EXTENSION

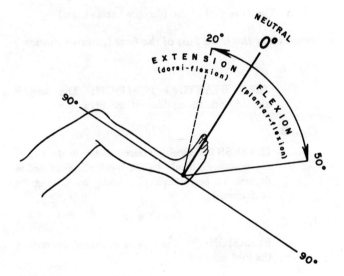

THE FOOT

HIND PART OF FOOT
(Passive Motion)

Motion of the foot is compound but can be broken down as—

1. The Hind part of the foot (the subtalar joint)
2. The Fore part of the foot (midtarsal joints)

Motions of the Hind Part of the Foot (passive motion):

Fig. A

> ZERO STARTING POSITION: The heel is aligned with the midline of the tibia.

Fig. B

> INVERSION: Heel is grasped firmly in the cup of the examiner's hand. Passive motion is estimated in degrees, or percentages of motion, by turning the heel inward.

Fig. C

> EVERSION: This motion is estimated by turning the heel outward.

HIND PART of the FOOT (PASSIVE MOTION)

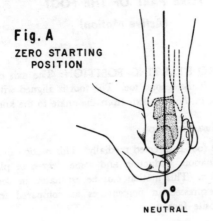

Fig. A
ZERO STARTING
POSITION

0°
NEUTRAL

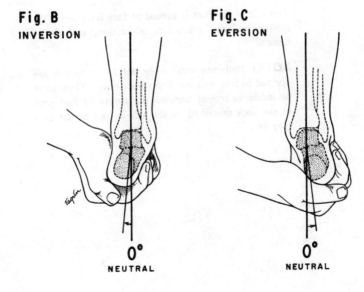

Fig. B
INVERSION

0°
NEUTRAL

Fig. C
EVERSION

0°
NEUTRAL

THE FOOT

FORE PART OF THE FOOT

(Active Motion)

Fig. A

ZERO STARTING POSITION: The axis of the foot is the second toe. The foot is aligned with the tibia in the long axis from the ankle to the knee.

Fig. B Active Inversion:

The foot is directed medially. This motion includes supination, adduction and some degree of plantar flexion. This motion can be estimated in degrees, or expressed in percentages as compared to the opposite foot.

Fig. C Active Eversion:

The sole of the foot is turned to face laterally. This motion includes pronation, abduction, and dorsiflexion.

NOTE: Problems exist when the foot motions are divided in fore and hindfoot descriptions. Care must be made to record motions pertaining to that part of the foot described or the whole foot as the case may be.

FORE PART of the FOOT

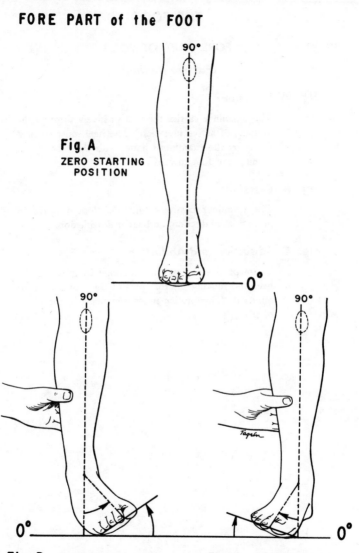

Fig. A
ZERO STARTING
POSITION

90°

0°

90°

90°

0°

0°

Fig. B INVERSION
(SUPINATION, ADDUCTION)
AND PLANTAR FLEXION

Fig. C EVERSION
(PRONATION, ABDUCTION)
AND DORSI-FLEXION

THE FOOT

FORE PART OF FOOT
(Passive Motion)

Fig. A Inversion:

The examiner carries the foot passively through the motions of active inversion. The heel must be held firmly by the examiner's hand, with the other hand turning the foot inward.

Fig. B Eversion:

The examiner passively turns the foot outward in pronation, abduction, and slight dorsiflexion.

Fig. C Adduction and Abduction:

These passive motions are obtained by grasping the heel and moving the fore part of the foot inward or outward. This motion must take place in the plane of the sole of the foot.

FORE PART of the FOOT

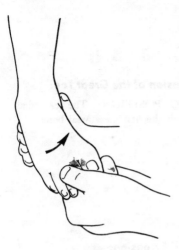

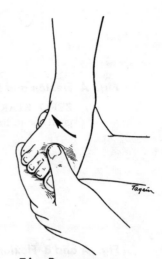

Fig. A INVERSION

Fig. B EVERSION

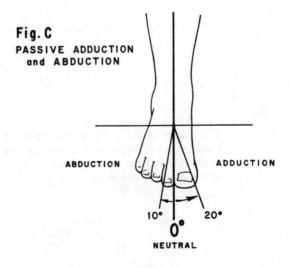

Fig. C
PASSIVE ADDUCTION
and ABDUCTION

ABDUCTION

ADDUCTION

10°   20°

0°

NEUTRAL

THE GREAT TOE

Fig. A Flexion and Extension of the Great Toe:

ZERO STARTING POSITION: The extended great toe in line with the first metatarsal bone.

Fig. A and B Flexion and Extension:

Is present at the metatarsophalangeal joint, and flexion only at the interphalangeal joint.

Fig. C

The degree of deformity of the great toe in this instance, hallux valgus, may be measured in degrees of abduction of the metatarsal bone, and adduction of the proximal and distal phalanges.

THE GREAT TOE

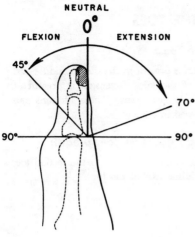

Fig. A METATARSOPHALANGEAL JOINT

NEUTRAL
0°

FLEXION EXTENSION

45°

70°

90° 90°

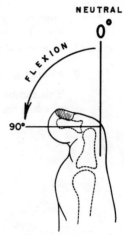

Fig. B INTERPHALANGEAL JOINT

NEUTRAL
0°

FLEXION

90°

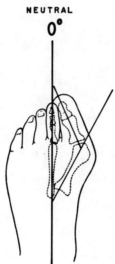

Fig. C
HALLUX VALGUS

NEUTRAL
0°

THE TOES

Fig. A Second to Fifth Toes:

Motion in flexion is present in the distal, middle and proximal joint of the toes. Extension is present at the metatarsophalangeal joint. These motions can be simply expressed in degrees.

Fig. B Abduction and Adduction (toe spread):

This can be measured in relation to the second toe, which is the midline axis of the foot.

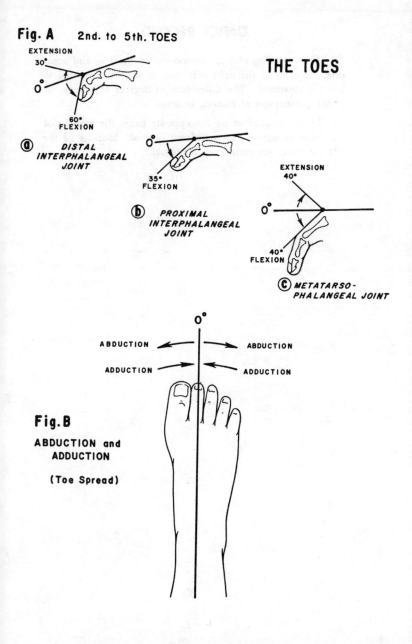

Fig. A 2nd. to 5th. TOES

THE TOES

EXTENSION
30°
0°
60°
FLEXION

ⓐ DISTAL INTERPHALANGEAL JOINT

0°
35° FLEXION

ⓑ PROXIMAL INTERPHALANGEAL JOINT

EXTENSION
40°
0°
40° FLEXION

ⓒ METATARSO-PHALANGEAL JOINT

0°

ABDUCTION ← → ABDUCTION

ADDUCTION → ← ADDUCTION

Fig. B
ABDUCTION and ADDUCTION

(Toe Spread)

OFFICE RECORD

The recording of joint motion should be clear and accurate. Motions of the right extremity should be compared to the left extremity. The difference, in degrees of motion, or in the percentages of motion, is noted.

In the illustration on the opposite page, the motions of the right extremity are considered normal. Motions of the left extremity are considered abnormal.

SAMPLE OFFICE RECORD
(All figures are in degrees)

JOINT	(normal extremity) RIGHT	(abnormal extremity) LEFT
HIP =		
FLEXION	120 (0 to 120)	45
EXTENSION	30 (0 to 30)	15
ROTATION		
in flexion =		
int. rot.	45 (0 to 45)	0
ext. rot.	45 (0 to 45)	10
in extension =		
int. rot.	45 (0 to 45)	0
ext. rot.	45 (0 to 45)	10
ABDUCTION	50 (0 to 50)	10
ADDUCTION	40 (0 to 40)	5
TOTAL MOTION	420	95
ELBOW =		
FLEXION	135 (0 to 135)	30 to 90
WRIST =		
FLEXION	80	40
EXTENSION	70	35
ULNAR DEVIATION	20	10
RADIAL DEVIATION	30	15

ESTIMATES OF
AVERAGE RANGES OF JOINT MOTION

The average ranges of joint motion can not be accurately determined, due to the wide variation in the degrees of motion amongst individuals of varying physical build and age groups. The following estimates are to serve merely as a guide, and not as a standard. The patient's opposite extremity is perhaps the best "normal" standard. In those instances when the opposite extremity has been injured, or is not present, these figures may prove helpful. Four sources are used for references. An average of these estimates is given. The sources are as follows:

Column (1)

The Committee on Medical Rating of Physical Impairment, Journal American Medical Association (ref. 12).

Column (2)

The Committee of the California Medical Association and Industrial Accident Commission of the State of California (ref. 5).

Column (3)

A System of Joint Measurements, William A. Clarke, Mayo Clinic (ref. 3).

Column (4)

The Committee on Joint Motion, American Academy of Orthopaedic Surgeons.

AVERAGE RANGES OF JOINT MOTION

JOINT	SOURCES (1)	(2)	(3)	(4)	AVERAGES
ELBOW =					
FLEXION	150	135	150	150	146
HYPEREXTENSION	0	0	0	0	0
FOREARM =					
PRONATION	80	75	50	80	71
SUPINATION	80	85	90	80	84
WRIST =					
EXTENSION	60	65	90	70	71
FLEXION	70	70		80	73
ULNAR DEV.	30	40	30	30	33
RADIAL DEV.	20	20	15	20	19
THUMB =					
ABDUCTION		55	50	70	58
FLEXION					
I-P Jt.	80	75	90	80	81
M — P	60	50	50	50	53
M — C				15	15
EXTENSION					
Distal Jt.		20	10	20	17
M — P		5	10	0	8
M — C				20	20
FINGERS =					
FLEXION					
Distal Jt.	70	70	90	90	80
Middle Jt.	100	100		100	100
Proximal Jt.	90	90		90	90

AVERAGE RANGES OF JOINT MOTION

JOINT	SOURCES (1)	(2)	(3)	(4)	AVERAGES
FINGERS =					
EXTENSION					
Distal Jt.				0	0
Middle Jt.				0	0
Proximal Jt.			45	45	45
SHOULDER =					
FORWARD FLEXION	150	170	130	180	158
HORIZONTAL FLEXION				135	135
BACKWARD EXTENSION	40	30	80	60	53
ABDUCTION	150	170	180	180	170
ADDUCTION	30		45	75	50
ROTATION					
Arm at Side					
Int. Rot.	40	60	90	80	68
Ext. Rot.	90	80	40	60	68
Arm in Abduction (90°)					
Int. Rot.				70	70
Ext. Rot.				90	90
HIP =					
FLEXION	100	110	120	120	113
EXTENSION	30	30	20	30	28
ABDUCTION	40	50	55	45	48
ADDUCTION	20	30	45	30	31
ROTATION					
In Flexion =					
Int. Rot.				45	45
Ext. Rot.				45	45
In Extension =					
Int. Rot.	40	35	20	45	35
Ext. Rot.	50	50	45	45	48
ABDUCTION					
In 90° of flexion			45 to 60 (depending on age)		

AVERAGE RANGES OF JOINT MOTION
SOURCES

JOINT	(1)	(2)	(3)	(4)	AVERAGES
KNEE =					
FLEXION	120	135	145	135	134
HYPEREXTENSION			10	10	10
ANKLE =					
FLEXION (plantar flexion)	40	50	50	50	48
EXTENSION (dorsiflexion)	20	15	15	20	18
HIND FOOT (subtalar) =					
INVERSION				5	5
EVERSION				5	5
FORE FOOT =					
INVERSION	30	35		35	33
EVERSION	20	20		15	18
TOES =					
GREAT TOE I-P Jt.					
Flexion	30			90	60
Extension	0			0	0
Proximal Jt.					
Flexion	30	35		45	37
Extension	50	70		70	63
2nd TO 5th TOES =					
FLEXION					
Distal Jt.	50			60	55
Middle Jt.	40			35	38
Proximal Jt.	30			40	35
Extension	40			40	40

85

AVERAGE RANGES OF JOINT MOTION

SOURCES

JOINT	(1)	(2)	(3)	(4)	AVERAGES
SPINE =					
CERVICAL					
FLEXION	30			45	38
EXTENSION	30			45	38
LAT. BENDING	40			45	43
ROTATION	30			60	45
THORACIC AND LUMBAR					
FLEXION	90			{80 4″	{85 4″
EXTENSION	30			20-30	30
LAT. BENDING	20			35	28
ROTATION	30			45	38

REFERENCES

1   American Society for Surgery of The Hand, Personal Consultations 1960-1962.

2   Cave, E. F. & Roberts, S. M., "A Method of Measuring and Recording Joint Function." J. Bone & Joint Surg: 18:2:455 - 466: April 1936.

3   Clark, William A., "A System of Joint Measurements" The J. Orthopaedic Surgery Vol. 2: No. 12: Dec. 1920.

4   Codman, E. A., The Shoulder. T. Todd, Boston 1934.

5   Evaluation of Industrial Disability (Comm. of California Medical Asso. & The Industrial Acc. Comm. of the State of California) Oxford Univ. Press. 1960.

6   Executive Comm. of American Academy of Orthopaedic Surgeons: Sept. 12, 1959. (Executive Comm. Meeting).

7   Executive Comm. of American Orthopaedic Association: Jan. 1960. (Executive Comm. Meeting).

8   Fractures & Other Injuries — Cave, E. F., Yearbook Publishing Co., 1958, pg. 10-21.

9   Gardner, Gray, O'Rahilly Anatomy — W. B. Saunders, Phila. & London, 1960.

10 Glimcher, Melvin & Brown, Thornton, Dept. Biophysics, Mass. Institute of Technology, 1959.

11 Harris, R. I. — A Memorandum of Movements of Joints, 1918.

12 Journal American Medical Association — "A Guide to the Evaluation of Permanent Impairment of the Extremities & Back." Special Edition, pg. 1-112, Feb. 15, 1958.

13 "Outline of Treatment of Fractures" — American College of Surgeons, 7th Ed. 1960.

14 Solomon, Louis, Personal Communication, Johannesburg, S. A.

15 The United States Armed Forces Medical Journal: Vol 6, No. 3, March 1955, The Joint Motion Measurements— Dept. of the Army & The Air Force. T.M. 8-640: A.F.P. 160-14-1. Mar. 1956.

16 Workman's Compensation Board, Toronto, Canada, Form 43 & 149.

17 Combined meeting, Orthopaedic Associations of the English Speaking World, Vancouver, B.C., June 1964.